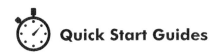 **Quick Start Guides**

The Essential
HEALTHY
SMOOTHIE
Recipe Book

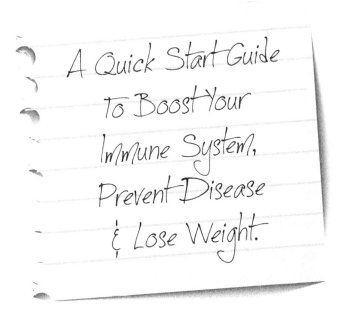

A Quick Start Guide To Boost Your Immune System, Prevent Disease & Lose Weight.

Delicious Smoothies For
Anti-Ageing, Energising & Detoxifying

First published in 2020 by Erin Rose Publishing

Text and illustration copyright © 2020 Erin Rose Publishing

Design: Julie Anson

ISBN: 978-1-9161523-6-6

A CIP record for this book is available from the British Library.

DISCLAIMER: his book is for informational purposes only and not intended as a substitute for the medical advice, diagnosis or treatment of a physician or qualified healthcare provider. The reader should consult a physician before undertaking a new health care regime and in all matters relating to his/her health, and particularly with respect to any symptoms that may require diagnosis or medical attention.

While every care has been taken in compiling the recipes for this book we cannot accept responsibility for any problems which arise as a result of preparing one of the recipes. The author and publisher disclaim responsibility for any adverse effects that may arise from the use or application of the recipes in this book. Some of the recipes in this book include nuts. If you have a nut allergy it's important to avoid these

CONTENTS

Introduction...1

Super Foods, Healthy Smoothies, Better Health 2

What You Need To Get Started 3

Helpful Tips To Make The Best Smoothies..4

Benefits Of Super Foods For Optimum Health 5

Smoothie Recipes

Mango & Cashew Protein Smoothie 10

Key Lime Pie Smoothie 11

Immune Boosting Sunrise Smoothie 12

Creamy Melon Hydrating Smoothie 13

Banana & Oat Smoothie..14

Beetroot & Strawberry Smoothie 15

Digestion Friendly Smoothie 16

Kefir & Berry Digestive Support Smoothie 17

Orange & Mango Refresher..18

Antioxidant Rich Matcha Smoothie 19

Tropical Mango & Passion Fruit Smoothie 20

Pomegranate and Blueberry Antioxidant Smoothie...............................21

Berry Rich Breakfast Smoothie...22

Pumpkin & Mango Vitamin Rich Smoothie...23

Cranberry & Blackcurrant Cleansing Smoothie 24

Mango, Apple & Mint Smoothie 25

Creamy Chocolate & Sweet Potato Smoothie..26

Creamy Lemon Cheesecake Smoothie..27

Strawberry, Quinoa & Chamomile Smoothie...28

Cherry & Coconut Water Smoothie 29

Nutty Chocolate Maca Smoothie 30

Glowing Skin Healthy Smoothie 31

Spiced Peach Smoothie 32

Nourishing Sweet Potato Smoothie 33

Mango & Sweet Potato Smoothie..34

Anti-Inflammatory Smoothie 35

Green Goodness Smoothie..36

Banana & Walnut Smoothie 37

Sirt Food Cocktail...38

Summer Berry Smoothie...39

Strawberry & Citrus Blend 40

Grapefruit & Celery Blast...41

Orange & Celery Crush 42

Tropical Chocolate Delight 43

Walnut & Spiced Apple Tonic...44

Pineapple & Cucumber Smoothie 45

Sweet Rocket Boost 46

Avocado, Celery & Pineapple Smoothie..47

Banana & Ginger Snap...48

Chocolate, Strawberry & Coconut Crush 49

Chocolate Berry Blend...50

Black Forest Smoothie...51

Creamy Coffee Smoothie..52

Acai Berry & Pineapple Smoothie 53

Creamy Strawberry & Orange Smoothie...54

Plum, Ginger & Beetroot Smoothie...55

Pineapple & Lime Smoothie...56

Wheatgrass, Lemon & Ginger Smoothie...57

Hydrating Apple, Coriander & Chilli Smoothie 58

Detox Wheatgrass & Beetroot Smoothie 59

Pear, Grape & Lucuma Smoothie...................................60

Lychee & Melon Smoothie...................................61

Mango, Celery & Ginger Smoothie...................................62

Orange, Carrot & Kale Smoothie...................................63

Creamy Strawberry & Cherry Smoothie 64

Cranberry & Kale Crush...................................65

Mango & Rocket (Arugula) Smoothie...................................66

Spiced Carrot Refresher...................................67

Berry & Carrot Smoothie...................................68

Coconut, Spinach & Lime Smoothie 69

Cleansing Cucumber Smoothie...................................70

Minty Lime Shots 71

Chocolate Protein Shake 72

Kiwi & Lettuce Shots 73

Pear Salad Smoothie 74

Avocado & Banana Smoothie...................................75

Pear & Cucumber Smoothie...................................76

Cucumber, Lemon & Coconut Refresher...................................77

Pink Grapefruit & Turmeric Smoothie 78

Peanut Butter & Banana Smoothie 79

Carrot & Celery Cleanser...................................80

Nutty Kale Smoothie 81

Tomato & Ginger Smoothie...................................82

Grapefruit & Carrot Smoothie...................................83

Coffee & Almond Smoothie...................................84

Banana & Coconut Smoothie 85

Basil Blackcurrant Refresher...................................86

Kiwi & Coconut Smoothie 87

Lush Green Smoothie...................................88

Apple, Spinach & Seed Smoothie 89

Coconut & Cucumber Smoothie 90

Green Detox Smoothie 91

Raspberry & Carrot Smoothie 92

Tomato & Carrot Smoothie 93

Apple & Grapefruit Smoothie 94

Cashew & Apricot Smoothie 95

Carrot & Apple Smoothie 96

Apple & Ginger Smoothie 97

Detox Smoothie 98

Carrot & Blackberry Smoothie 99

Kiwi Salad Smoothie 100

Blackberry & Carrot Smoothie 101

Coconut & Lemon Zinger 102

Creamy Raspberry Smoothie 103

INTRODUCTION

Boost your immunity, improve your health, reduce inflammation and lose weight naturally with easy and delicious smoothies. They are packed with vitamins and nutrients, fresh, easy-to-source ingredients which are filling, hydrating and full of goodness to boost your health and improve your vitality. Smoothies are a nutritious, tasty meal in a glass and they are so simple to make. Support and build a strong immune system with antioxidants to help your body fight off colds, flus and viruses and also deal with stress.

You can easily enjoy power-packed, one-step meals which keep you feeling full as they can contain protein, fibre and healthy fats. Smoothies can be tailored to your taste and needs, choosing frozen or fresh fruits, vegetables, yogurt, nuts, seeds, herbs and spices to suit you. A daily smoothie can help you kick-start and maintain healthy eating and you'll feel the benefits as you curb hunger cravings and begin to feel more energised.

A smoothie can be a quick snack, or a meal, prepared in minutes using a blender and a few simple ingredients. They are ideal for many dietary needs, including vegan, calorie-restriction, vegetarian, dairy and non-dairy, detox, elimination diets and simple healthy eating.

Creating luscious, creamy drinks is super-easy to do. You can use grains, nuts, seeds, dairy, cocoa power, nut butter, protein powder, coffee or digestive support and herbal supplements. Choose from a wide variety of recipes and experiment to find your favourite.

Choose from recipes which are light and refreshing like pineapple & cucumber or lemon cheesecake and chocolate berry blend to recipes which are digestion friendly, and can help promote healthy skin.

Enrich and fuel your body with quality nutrients to ward off pathogens, reduce free-radicals and help natural detoxification. Keep your immune system strong and enjoy having more energy while you lose weight.

Super Foods, Healthy Smoothies, Better Health

A plentiful supply of 'Superfood Smoothies' can boost your health. Superfoods are not magical foods, they are basically foods which are simply good for you, such as fruits and vegetables which are high in antioxidants, healthy fats, vitamins and minerals. They are natural foods which contain health boosting nutrients. Superfood is a modern term for natural foods and we recognise the need to fill our diets with good quality nutrients. Adding super-healthy, super-nutritious foods to smoothies is sure way to maximise the healing, health giving properties of nature's bountiful gifts for our best health and wellbeing.

Our immune systems thrive on nutrients from fruits, vegetables, helping us to stay strong and effectively fight off illness. A diet in vitamins, minerals and antioxidants helps us to stay in peak condition and if your diet has been lacking in good nutrients, adding smoothies to your diet will help overcome the effects of an unhealthy diet. It won't happen overnight but it will happen, especially when healthy smoothies are part of your usual diet.

Smoothies are so convenient! They require no cooking and very little preparation. Smoothie ingredients can be prepared in batches, divided into portions and stored in the freezer until you are ready to use them. There is a wide selection of frozen fruit and vegetables in the supermarkets, which are ideal for this purpose and still contain plenty of nutrients.

Superfood powders such as matcha, baobab, lucuma and protein powders are not necessary. You can start off with basic fruits and vegetables or you can buy in store cupboard ingredients, for variety, flavour and extra nutrition.

Making smoothies yourself you know there are no artificial sweeteners or added sugar in your drink. Concentrated fruit juices which can have a negative impact on the body due to the amount of fruit sugar and having much of the natural fibre removed.

When making smoothies however, the fibre is part of the drink which is not only good for your digestive system, it slows down the absorption of fructose (fruit sugar) in the body which is better for blood sugar levels.

What You Need To Get Started

Firstly, a good blender is top of the list. There are many blenders to choose from, in different price ranges and capacities. A personal blender will usually be enough for one person, often the jug part is suitable to drink from and has less parts to clean so they are simple and easy to use.

Some jug blenders have many attachments and require more cleaning, although they may have a larger capacity for families. The power of the blender is also an important factor, for instance, can it crush ice cubes and blend firm fruit and vegetables to a smooth consistency.

So size, speed, ease of use and cleaning are all things to consider. If you are just starting out making smoothies you may not wish to invest too much money into a blender just yet but you don't want to be put off by a blender which creates a lot of mess and fuss and gives you smoothies which aren't smooth.

High performance blenders may cost more than budget blenders however bullet type blenders tend to do the job and not cost to much and they are a popular choice.

What fruits, vegetables and flavours do you enjoy most? Start stocking up with these and keep a good supply in your fridge, freezer or store cupboard. The benefits of organic produce are not just that they contain less pesticides and chemicals but they are also richer in nutrients too – not to mention some find they also taste so much better.

Helpful Tips To Create The Best Smoothies

If your smoothie becomes too thin you can add some banana or frozen fruit to give it a thicker, creamier texture.

Frozen bananas are a great addition to a smoothie, so if you have very ripe bananas which could spoil you can freeze them to use later. Remove the skin first, chop them and divide into portions if you like. You can also do this with other fruits to avoid waste.

You can save time on preparation by chopping fruit and popping it into freezer bags in individual portions.

Powerful blenders generally have no problem crushing nuts (or ice) however if yours leaves them lumpy you can add nut butter instead and bypass the need for the blender to do it.

If tough leafy veggies like kale don't come out well blended you can try blending them with a little water first, then adding it to the final blend.

Ingredients like melon and cucumber contain a lot of water already so you may wish to add less liquid to smoothies containing them, so you can keep the texture creamy and the flavour stronger.

To get the right consistency you can start off with less liquid and increase it until you reach the desired thickness. If you wish to avoid dairy milk, you can try a wide range of alternatives, such as almond, rice, hazelnut, soya or coconut milk. Or you can add green tea, juices or coconut water.

When a smoothie lacks sweetness, which can be the case in green leafy smoothies especially, try adding pineapple, banana or strawberry to counteract the bitterness. Although strawberry may give a green smoothie a slightly unappealing brown tinge it can do wonders for the flavour.

There are a wide range or protein powders on the market with everything from whey protein, to soya or pea protein which is ideal for anyone on a vegan diet. As well as providing extra protein they can also add sweetness. Start off with a little and increase according to taste as some protein powders are incredibly sweet.

For extra creaminess, a lovely ripe avocado will enrich your smoothie and provide you with delicious healthy fats. Alternatively, you can try natural yogurt, coconut yogurt, coconut milk, kefir, milk or dairy-free milk alternatives.

Tastes change, especially when we change our eating habits and choose healthier options and some smoothies may begin to taste too sweet. In which case, try adding a squeeze of lemon or lime juice.

If you are adding ice to a smoothie, be mindful that a lot of ice can dilute the flavour, so adjust the amount to suit you or you can leave it out altogether.

Benefits Of Super Foods For Optimum Health

We're often bombarded with news of what is healthy and what is not which can be overwhelming. Yet natural wholefoods foods are guaranteed to be full of nutrients and not just a fad. So here are some top plant-based foods which will have a positive impact on your health.

Almonds
Almonds are full of protein, zinc, vitamin E, magnesium, iron, fibre and B vitamins. Choosing organic, where possible will help you avoid any heavily sprayed nuts. They are so versatile and also contain calcium. Almond butter or almond milk makes a great staple for your store cupboard. They contain healthy fats and are good for blood sugar, cholesterol, weight loss and improve gut bacteria.

Apples
Packed with vitamin C they are great antioxidants and boost the immune system. They contain pectin which is a type of fibre which is good for cholesterol, the colon, digestion, prostate and blood sugar levels.

Avocados
Avocados are best known for being a rich source of healthy fats but they also contain many other nutrients, such as vitamins C, E, K, folate, riboflavin, magnesium, niacin, pantothenic acid and potassium. Don't avoid them because

of the fat, they are essential fatty acids and good for you. They are good for heart disease, cholesterol, skin, hair, hormone balance and libido.

Bananas
Bananas are a good source of potassium and are known to be beneficial for blood pressure and digestion too due to their fibre and vitamin C content. They are neatly packed and make a handy energy boosting snack. They are good for the immune system, skin, nervous system and weight loss.

Blueberries
Blueberries are a 'sirtfood' as they contain 'sirtuins' which is a compound which boosts metabolism, improves weight loss, longevity and cell function. These really are worth adding to your diet! Blueberries are a rich source of antioxidants and polyphenols which help regulate insulin production and improve blood sugar levels.

Cacao (cocoa)
Cocoa is also a sirtfood which is not only delicious but can enhance weight loss. Unfortunately lots of added sugar in chocolate bars negates the positive benefits of cocoa. You can add 100% cocoa powder or cacao into your smoothies and enjoy its antioxidant properties, iron and magnesium content. It also enhances the mood and helps with muscle and nerve function.

Coconut
Coconut water is a good source of potassium which makes it good for blood pressure and the heart, plus it's hydrating. Coconut is rich in protein and it's a satiating, digestive-friendly fibre which is great for the colon. It can improve weight loss and build muscle while improving fatigue and constipation. Coconut oil is a source of healthy fats for skin and hair.

Celery
Celery contains vitamin C, beta carotene, flavonoids and antioxidants so it's great to protect the cells and helps ward off disease. It's good for gut health, digestion and bowel regularity. It has a high water content and is diuretic so it's great for

reducing fluid retention in the body. Its powerful flavour can make it unsuitable for some smoothies but adding a small piece can give your smoothie an extra boost.

Ginger
Ginger is widely used for nausea and digestive upsets, motion sickness and dizziness. Its warming properties give smoothies a bite and added to hot water and lemon to help fight off colds. It's used in traditional remedies for morning sickness plus it contains vitamin C, iron, zinc, magnesium and potassium. Research shows it has a beneficial effect on blood sugar in pre-diabetes.

Kale
Kale is one of the most nutrient dense foods. It is packed with vitamins A, C, K and manganese and as it is very high in antioxidants it is useful for protecting the body from free-radical damage. It can help support the immune system, improve constipation, blood clotting, eyes, weight loss and healthy bones. Kale is a greatly nutritious for the whole body.

Sweet Potatoes
Sweet potatoes are rich in vitamins, minerals and fibre. It is also rich in beta-carotene and may help protect against cancer, plus it's beneficial for eye health. The nutrients in sweet potatoes can help boost immunity, reduce inflammation and obesity.

Lemon
Lemons are high in vitamin C and pectin which could explain why it is considered beneficial for weight loss as pectin aids digestion and bowel function. Because of the high vitamin C content they can aid the absorption of iron in the body.

Linseeds (Flaxseeds)
Linseeds are a rich source of omega-3 fatty acids. It could help with cholesterol and cardiovascular disease. It's very useful for anyone suffering from constipation of digestive trouble as well as that some research shows it can be used for inflammation and arthritis. It's worth giving it a shot.

Oats

Oats are known for improving cholesterol levels. balancing blood sugar, promoting good digestion and providing beta-glucan, antioxidants, vitamins and minerals. This simple food also helps with constipation, weight loss, providing fibre and promoting healthy gut bacteria. They really are well-worth adding to your daily diet.

Oranges

Oranges are high in vitamin C which makes them useful in preventing anaemia and helping with iron absorption. They are also a good source of fibre, potassium and antioxidants. Oranges are good for youthful looking skin, collagen, wound healing, and blood pressure. High amounts of vitamin C are also useful in inhibiting diseases such as cancer, aiding gut health, insulin levels, fatigue and inflammation.

Pineapple

Pineapples are deliciously exotic and they contain the enzyme bromelain which aids digestion, assists with inflammation and wound healing. It is also rich in vitamin C for healthy cell growth, manganese for healthy bone development. They contain flavonoids, and phenolics which are antioxidants which fight free radical damage which can cause, heart disease, Alzheimer's, inflammation and cancer.

Walnuts

Walnuts contain biotin which makes them a good choice for hair and nail growth. They contain healthy oils and fatty acids which help with healthy blood vessels, inflammation and cardiovascular health. The omega 3 and omega 6 contents makes them useful for motor function, depression and memory. They are a rich source of magnesium, calcium, iron potassium and folate. Add them into your diet for healthy skin, reproductive system and a good energy boost.

SMOOTHIE RECIPES

Mango & Cashew Protein Smoothie

SERVES 1

521 calories per serving

Ingredients

50g (2oz) unsalted cashew nuts

350mls (12fl oz) cold water

1 medium mango, stone and skin removed

1 tablespoon chia seeds (or linseeds)

1 tablespoon porridge oats

A few ice cubes

A little chopped mango for garnish

Method

Soak the cashew nuts overnight in a little water. In the morning, drain off the excess water and blitz them in a food processor with the 350mls (12fl oz) cold water. Add all the other ingredients and blend until smooth and creamy. Garnish with some chopped mango and drink straight away.

Key Lime Pie Smoothie

Ingredients

50g (2oz) desiccated (shredded) coconut (plus extra for garnish)

3 dates, pitted

1 small handful fresh spinach leaves

½ avocado, stone and skin removed

450mls (1 pint) chilled coconut water

Juice of 2 limes

A few ice cubes

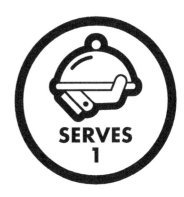

SERVES 1

597 calories per serving

Method

Place all of the ingredients into a blender and blitz until smooth and creamy. Serve in a tall glass and garnish with a sprinkling of coconut. Drink straight away.

Immune Boosting Sunrise Smoothie

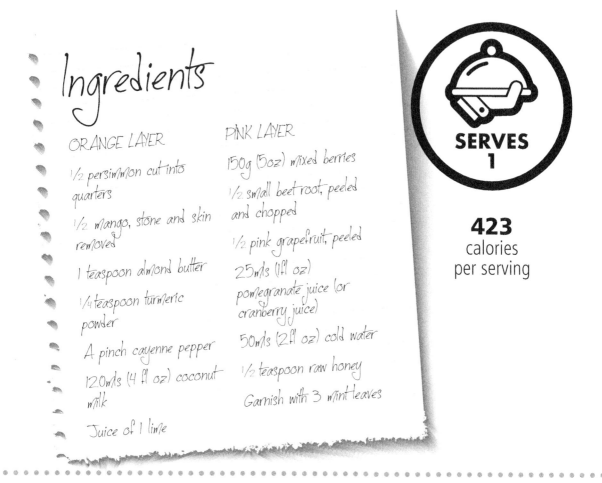

Ingredients

ORANGE LAYER

½ persimmon cut into quarters

½ mango, stone and skin removed

1 teaspoon almond butter

¼ teaspoon turmeric powder

A pinch cayenne pepper

120mls (4 fl oz) coconut milk

Juice of 1 lime

PINK LAYER

150g (5oz) mixed berries

½ small beetroot, peeled and chopped

½ pink grapefruit, peeled

25mls (1fl oz) pomegranate juice (or cranberry juice)

50mls (2fl oz) cold water

½ teaspoon raw honey

Garnish with 3 mint leaves

SERVES 1

423 calories per serving

Method

Place all of the ingredients for the orange layer into the blender and process until smooth. Pour it into a large glass. Add the ingredients for the pink layer into the blender and process until smooth. Pour this mixture on top of the orange layer. Garnish with some mint leaves.

Creamy Melon Hydrating Smoothie

Ingredients

150g fresh honeydew melon, seed removed and chopped

240mls (½ pint) almond milk

A few ice cubes

SERVES 1

97 calories per serving

Method

Place all of the ingredients into a blender and process until smooth. Enjoy straight away.

Banana & Oat Smoothie

SERVES 1

422
calories
per serving

Ingredients

50g (2oz) oats

1 medium banana, peeled

1 teaspoon almond butter

1/2 teaspoon cinnamon

1/2 teaspoon ground turmeric

1/2 teaspoon Himalayan salt

120mls (4fl oz) almond milk

Method

Place all of the ingredients into a blender and blitz until smooth and creamy. Enjoy!

Beetroot & Strawberry Smoothie

Ingredients

150g (5oz) strawberries

1/4 little gem lettuce

1/2 beetroot, peeled, diced

2.5cm (1 inch) piece of fresh ginger, peeled

A few cubes of ice

SERVES 1

81 calories per serving

Method

Place all of the ingredients into a blender and process until smooth. Ice can be added in during blending or if your machine isn't suitable you can add them to the glass. Serve immediately and enjoy!

Digestion Friendly Smoothie

Ingredients

SERVES 1

374 calories per serving

- 25g (1oz) oats
- 2.5cm (1 inch) chunk of fresh ginger, chopped finely and peeled
- 1 banana, peeled
- 1 tablespoon peanut butter
- 1 teaspoon of ground turmeric
- 1 teaspoon of hemp powder
- 1 teaspoon of chia seeds
- 240mls (½ pint) almond milk
- Pinch of black pepper

Method

Place all of the ingredients into a blender and process until smooth. Serve and enjoy.

Kefir & Berry Digestive Support Smoothie

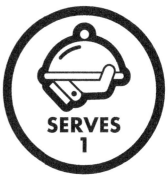

SERVES 1

421
calories
per serving

Ingredients

1 medium banana, peeled

75g (3oz) mixed frozen berries

25g (1oz) ground almonds

2 teaspoons honey

180mls (6fl oz) kefir

Method

Place all of the ingredients into a blender and blitz until smooth and creamy. Garnish it with a frozen berry or two and enjoy straight away.

Orange & Mango Refresher

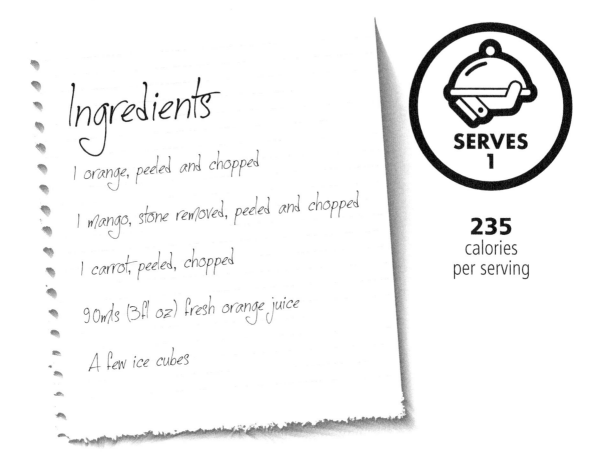

Ingredients

1 orange, peeled and chopped

1 mango, stone removed, peeled and chopped

1 carrot, peeled, chopped

90mls (3fl oz) fresh orange juice

A few ice cubes

SERVES 1

235 calories per serving

Method

Place all of the ingredients into a blender and process until smooth. Serve immediately and enjoy!

Antioxidant Rich Matcha Smoothie

Ingredients

150g (5oz) strawberries, hulled

1 scoop vanilla protein powder

1 handful of fresh spinach leaves

1 medium banana, peeled

½ teaspoon matcha powder

240mls (8fl oz) almond milk (or other milk)

A few ice cubes

SERVES 1

292 calories per serving

Method

Place all of the ingredients into a blender and blitz until smooth.

Tropical Mango & Passion Fruit Smoothie

Ingredients

125g (4oz) fresh mango flesh

1 medium banana, peeled

1 tablespoon linseeds (flaxseeds)

Seeds of 1 passion fruit

240mls (8fl oz) reduced fat coconut milk

SERVES 1

418 calories per serving

Method

Place the mango, banana, sunflower/linseeds and coconut milk into a blender and process until creamy. Pour it into a glass and add some passion fruit seeds on top. Enjoy straight away.

Pomegranate and Blueberry Antioxidant Smoothie

Ingredients

100g (3½ oz) blueberries

1 pomegranate, seeds only

1 tablespoon natural yogurt (optional)

1 tablespoon linseeds (flaxseeds)

1 teaspoon 100% cocoa or cacao nibs

A small handful of fresh kale, chopped

SERVES 1

253 calories per serving

Method

Place the ingredients into a blender with just enough water to cover them and process until smooth. Serve into a glass and add a sprinkle of cocoa powder to garnish.

Berry Rich Breakfast Smoothie

Ingredients

100g (3½ oz) blueberries

100g (3½ oz) raspberries

1 tablespoon porridge oats

1 tablespoon natural yogurt

1 tablespoon linseeds (flaxseeds)

240mls (½ pint) almond milk (or other milk)

SERVES 1

285
calories
per serving

Method

Place all of the ingredients into a blender and mix until smooth and creamy. Enjoy.

Pumpkin & Mango Vitamin Rich Smoothie

Ingredients

100g (3½ oz) pumpkin flesh

1 mango, stone and skin removed

1 medium banana, peeled

1 tablespoon linseeds

1 teaspoon honey (optional)

240mls (½ pint almond milk (or other milk)

SERVES 1

370 calories per serving

Method

Place all of the ingredients into a blender and blitz until creamy. Drink straight away.

Cranberry & Blackcurrant Cleansing Smoothie

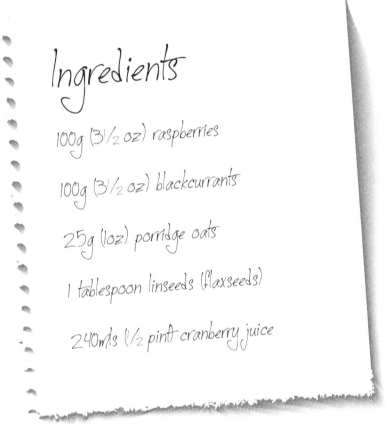

Ingredients

100g (3½ oz) raspberries

100g (3½ oz) blackcurrants

25g (1oz) porridge oats

1 tablespoon linseeds (flaxseeds)

240mls (½ pint) cranberry juice

SERVES 1

245 calories per serving

Method

Place all of the ingredients into a blender and process until smooth. You can adjust the taste and consistency with some extra cranberry juice. Enjoy.

Mango, Apple & Mint Smoothie

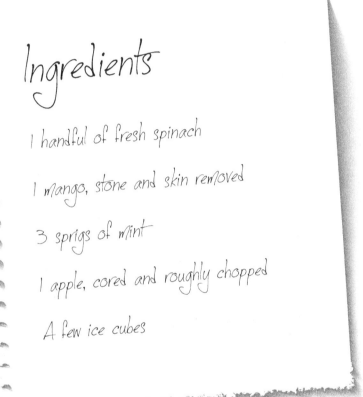

Ingredients

1 handful of fresh spinach

1 mango, stone and skin removed

3 sprigs of mint

1 apple, cored and roughly chopped

A few ice cubes

SERVES 1

178
calories
per serving

Method

Place all of the ingredients into a blender with enough water to cover it. Blitz until smooth and garnish with a little mint.

Creamy Chocolate & Sweet Potato Smoothie

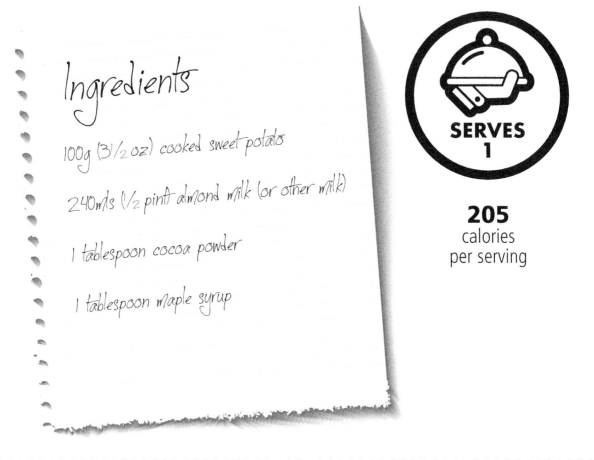

Ingredients

100g (3½ oz) cooked sweet potato

240mls (½ pint) almond milk (or other milk)

1 tablespoon cocoa powder

1 tablespoon maple syrup

SERVES 1

205 calories per serving

Method

Place all of the ingredients into a blender and process until smooth. Sprinkle with a little cocoa powder to garnish. Enjoy.

Creamy Lemon Cheesecake Smoothie

Ingredient

150g (5oz) mango flesh
50g (2oz) cooked chickpeas (garbanzo beans)
25g (1oz) chopped pecan nuts
1 medjool dates
Juice and zest of 1 medium lemon
¼ teaspoon ground turmeric
¼ teaspoon salt
240mls (½ pint) reduced fat coconut milk

SERVES 1

566
calories
per serving

Method

Place all of the ingredients into a blender and blitz until smooth and creamy. If it's too zesty, you can add a teaspoon of honey to sweeten the smoothie. You can also add a little water or extra coconut milk if you prefer a thinner texture. The chickpeas (garbanzo beans) give this smoothie a protein boost. Enjoy.

Strawberry, Quinoa & Chamomile Smoothie

Ingredients

180mls (6fl oz) chamomile tea

180mls (6fl oz) almond milk (or other milk)

75g (3oz) cooked quinoa (or oats)

200g (7oz) strawberries (fresh or frozen)

SERVES 1

186 calories per serving

Method

Place all of the ingredients into a blender and process until smooth and creamy. You can serve with chopped strawberry on top. Enjoy.

Cherry & Coconut Water Smoothie

Ingredients

200g (7oz) cherries (stone removed)

1 large banana, peeled

240mls (8fl oz) coconut water

SERVES 1

185
calories
per serving

Method

Place all of the ingredients into a blender and blitz until smooth.

Nutty Chocolate Maca Smoothie

Ingredients

240mls (½ pint) almond milk

150g (5oz) strawberries, hulled

25g (1oz) ground almonds

25g (1oz) chocolate maca or plant protein powder

14g (approx. ½ oz) organic hemp seed powder

25g (1oz) cacao nibs

SERVES 1

490 calories per serving

Method

Place all of the ingredients into a blender and process until smooth and creamy. Garnish with chopped strawberries or some seeds.

Glowing Skin Healthy Smoothie

Ingredients

150g (5oz) mango flesh
50g (2oz) cashew nuts
1 medium banana, peeled
2.5cm (1 inch) chunk of fresh ginger (peeled)
1 large medjool date
1 tablespoon chia seeds
1/2 teaspoon ground cardamom
1/4 teaspoon ground turmeric
240mls (8fl oz) coconut water

SERVES 1

568
calories
per serving

Method

Soak the cashew nuts in water for 30 minutes then add them to the blender. Add in the remaining ingredients and process until smooth. Garnish with a sprinkle of cardamom and/or turmeric and enjoy straight away.

Spiced Peach Smoothie

SERVES 1

240
calories
per serving

Ingredients

2 ripe peaches, stones removed

2.5cm (1 inch) chunk of fresh ginger

1 medium banana, peeled

1/4 teaspoon cinnamon

180mls (6fl oz) almond milk (or other milk)

1 tablespoon maple syrup (optional)

A few ice cubes

Method

Place all of the ingredients into the blender and process until smooth. Sprinkle with a little cinnamon to garnish.

Nourishing Sweet Potato Smoothie

Ingredients

75g (3oz) cooked sweet potato (leftovers are fine)

1 medium banana, peeled

1 teaspoon peanut butter

1 large medjool date

1/4 teaspoon ground turmeric

1/4 teaspoon ground cinnamon

1/4 teaspoon ground ginger or 1cm (roughly 1/2 inch) chunk of fresh ginger, peeled

180mls (6fl oz) almond milk (or other milk)

Pinch of salt

SERVES 1

271
calories
per serving

Method

Add all of the ingredient to a blender and blitz until smooth and creamy. You can add a little extra almond or other milk to adapt the consistency to your liking. Garnish with a sprinkle of cinnamon.

Mango & Sweet Potato Smoothie

Ingredients

75g (3oz) cooked sweet potato (leftovers are fine)

75g (3oz) mango flesh, stone and skin removed

1 tablespoon chia seeds

1 teaspoon honey

60mls (2fl oz) reduced fat coconut milk

A few ice cubes (optional)

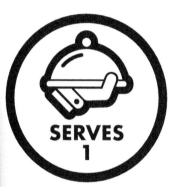

SERVES 1

252 calories per serving

Method

Place all of the ingredients into a blender and blitz until smooth. Enjoy straight away.

Anti-Inflammatory Smoothie

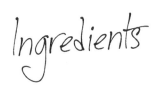

Ingredients

1 large handful fresh spinach leaves

1 cucumber, chopped

1 pear, cored

Juice of 1 lime

1 tablespoon chia seeds

A few ice cubes

SERVES 1

176
calories
per serving

Method

Place all of the ingredients into a blender and process until smooth. Enjoy.

Green Goodness Smoothie

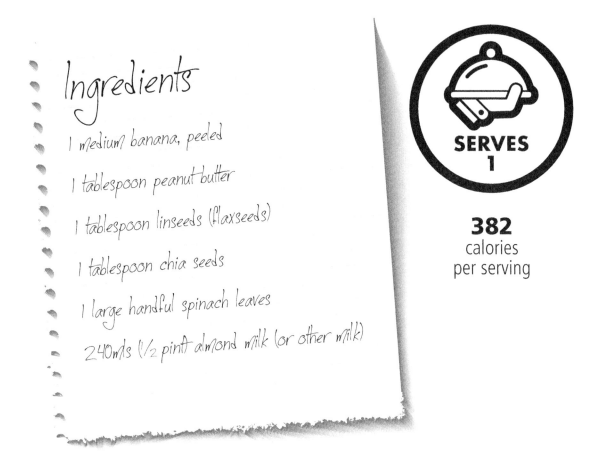

Ingredients

1 medium banana, peeled

1 tablespoon peanut butter

1 tablespoon linseeds (flaxseeds)

1 tablespoon chia seeds

1 large handful spinach leaves

240mls (½ pint) almond milk (or other milk)

SERVES 1

382 calories per serving

Method

Place all of the ingredients into a blender and process until smooth and creamy. If it isn't sweet enough, try adding a date or a little honey.

Banana & Walnut Smoothie

Ingredients

25g (1oz) oats

1 pitted date

1 medium banana, peeled

1 tablespoon chopped walnuts

1/4 teaspoon ground cinnamon

1/8 teaspoon ground nutmeg

1/2 teaspoon vanilla extract

180mls (6fl oz) almond milk (or other milk)

SERVES 1

336
calories
per serving

Method

Place all of the ingredients into a blender and process until smooth. Add an extra date if you prefer it sweeter. Serve and enjoy.

Sirt Food Cocktail

Ingredients

- 75g (3oz) kale
- 50g (2oz) strawberries
- 1 apple, cored
- 2 sticks of celery
- 1 tablespoon parsley
- 1 teaspoon of matcha powder
- Squeeze lemon juice (optional) to taste

SERVES 1

101 calories per serving

Method

Place the ingredients into a blender and add enough water to cover the ingredients and blitz to a smooth consistency.

Summer Berry Smoothie

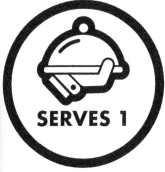

SERVES 1

146
calories
per serving

Ingredients

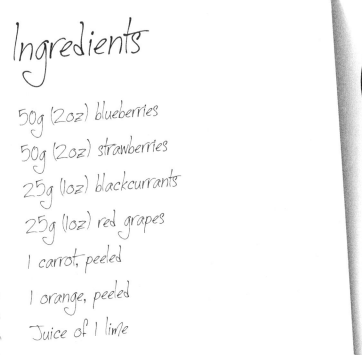

50g (2oz) blueberries

50g (2oz) strawberries

25g (1oz) blackcurrants

25g (1oz) red grapes

1 carrot, peeled

1 orange, peeled

Juice of 1 lime

Method

Place all of the ingredients into a blender and cover them with water. Blitz until smooth.
You can also add some crushed ice and a mint leaf to garnish.

Strawberry & Citrus Blend

Ingredients

75g (3oz) strawberries

1 apple, cored

1 orange, peeled

1/2 avocado, peeled and de-stoned

1/2 teaspoon matcha powder

Juice of 1 lime

**SERVES
1**

272
calories
per serving

Method

Place all of the ingredients into a blender with enough water to cover them and process until smooth.

Grapefruit & Celery Blast

Ingredients

1 grapefruit, peeled

2 stalks of celery

1/2 teaspoon matcha powder

SERVES 1

70 calories per serving

Method

Place all the ingredients into a blender with enough water to cover them and blitz until smooth.

Orange & Celery Crush

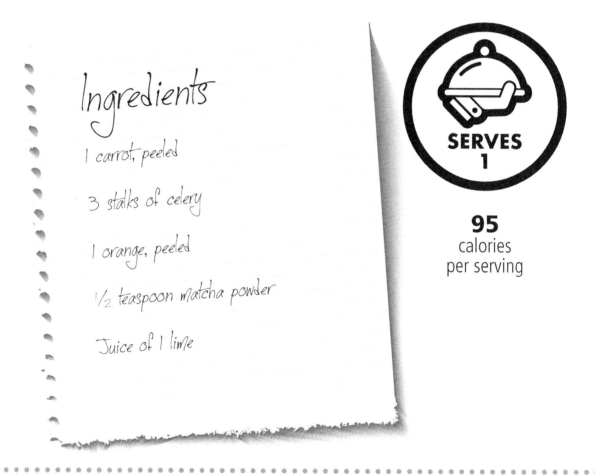

Ingredients

1 carrot, peeled

3 stalks of celery

1 orange, peeled

1/2 teaspoon matcha powder

Juice of 1 lime

SERVES 1

95 calories per serving

Method

Place all of the ingredients into a blender with enough water to cover them and blitz until smooth.

Tropical Chocolate Delight

Ingredients

1 mango, skin and stone removed

75g (3oz) fresh pineapple, chopped

1 tablespoon 100% cocoa powder or cacao nibs

150mls (5fl oz) coconut milk

A small handful of kale or spinach (optional)

SERVES 1

420
calories
per serving

Method

Place all of the ingredients into a blender and blitz until smooth. You can add a little water if it seems too thick.

Walnut & Spiced Apple Tonic

Ingredients

6 walnuts halves

1 apple, cored

1 medium banana, peeled

1/2 teaspoon matcha powder

1/2 teaspoon cinnamon

Pinch of ground nutmeg

SERVES 1

272 calories per serving

Method

Place all of the ingredients into a blender and add sufficient water to cover them. Blitz until smooth and creamy.

Pineapple & Cucumber Smoothie

Ingredients

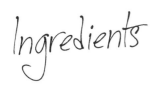

50g (2oz) cucumber

1 stalk of celery

2 slices of fresh pineapple

2 sprigs of parsley

½ teaspoon matcha powder

Squeeze of lemon juice

SERVES 1

77
calories
per serving

Method

Place all of the ingredients into blender with enough water to cover them and blitz until smooth.

45

Sweet Rocket Boost

SERVES 1

113
calories
per serving

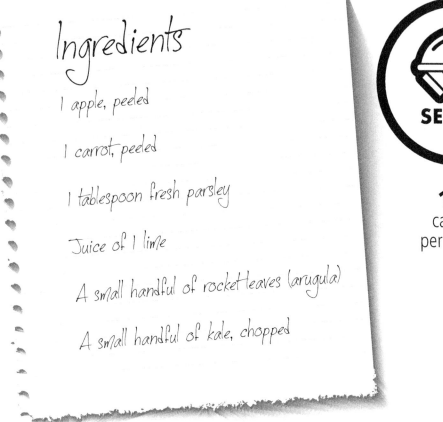

Ingredients

1 apple, peeled

1 carrot, peeled

1 tablespoon fresh parsley

Juice of 1 lime

A small handful of rocket leaves (arugula)

A small handful of kale, chopped

Method

Place all of the ingredients into a blender with enough water to cover and process until smooth

Avocado, Celery & Pineapple Smoothie

Ingredients

SERVES 1

306
calories
per serving

50g (2oz) fresh pineapple, peeled and chopped

3 stalks of celery

1 avocado, peeled & de-stoned

1 teaspoon fresh parsley

½ teaspoon matcha powder

Juice of ½ lemon

Method

Place all of the ingredients into a blender and add enough water to cover them. Process until creamy and smooth.

Banana & Ginger Snap

Ingredients

1 medium banana, peeled

1 large carrot, peeled

1 apple, cored

1/2 stick of celery

1/4 level teaspoon turmeric powder

2.5cm (1 inch) chunk of fresh ginger, peeled

SERVES 1

166 calories per serving

Method

Place all the ingredients into a blender with just enough water to cover them. Process until smooth.

Chocolate, Strawberry & Coconut Crush

Ingredients

100mls (3½ fl oz) coconut milk

100g (3½ oz) strawberries

1 medium banana, peeled

1 tablespoon 100% cocoa powder or cacao nibs

1 teaspoon matcha powder

SERVES 1

324
calories
per serving

Method

Toss all of the ingredients into a blender and process them to a creamy consistency. Add a little extra water if you need to thin it a little.

Chocolate Berry Blend

Ingredients

50g (2oz) blueberries

50g (2oz) strawberries

1 banana, peeled

1 tablespoon 100% cocoa powder or cacao nibs

200mls (7fl oz) unsweetened soya milk

A small handful of kale

SERVES 1

241 calories per serving

Method

Place all of the ingredients into a blender with enough water to cover them and process until smooth.

Black Forest Smoothie

Ingredients

100g (3½ oz) frozen cherries

1 medjool date

1 tablespoon cocoa powder

2 teaspoons chia seeds

200mls (7fl oz) almond milk (or other milk alternative)

A small handful of fresh spinach (optional)

SERVES 1

337
calories
per serving

Method

Place all the ingredients into a blender and process until smooth and creamy.

Creamy Coffee Smoothie

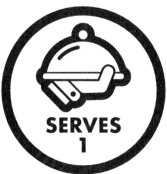

SERVES 1

239 calories per serving

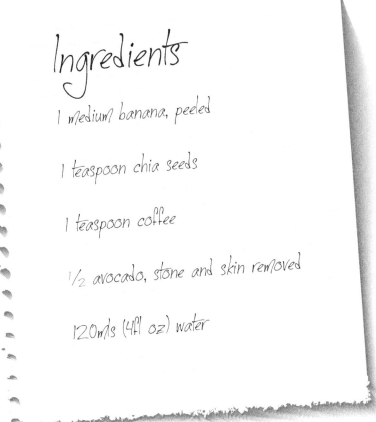

Ingredients

1 medium banana, peeled

1 teaspoon chia seeds

1 teaspoon coffee

1/2 avocado, stone and skin removed

120mls (4fl oz) water

Method

Place all the ingredients into a food processor or blender and blitz until smooth. You can add a little crushed ice too. This can also double as a breakfast smoothie.

Acai Berry & Pineapple Smoothie

Ingredients

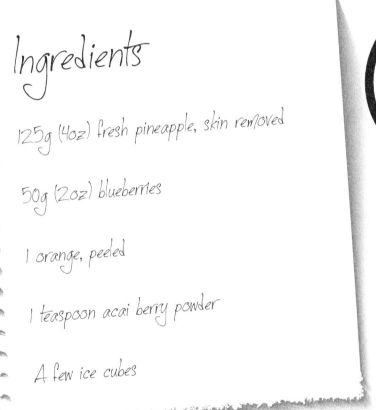

125g (4oz) fresh pineapple, skin removed

50g (2oz) blueberries

1 orange, peeled

1 teaspoon acai berry powder

A few ice cubes

SERVES 1

153
calories
per serving

Method

Place all of the ingredients into a blender and add just enough water to cover the ingredients. Blitz until smooth. Enjoy.

Creamy Strawberry & Orange Smoothie

Ingredients

150g (5oz) strawberries, hulled

1 pear, cored

1 orange, peeled

1 tablespoon reduced fat coconut milk

A few drops of vanilla extract

240mls (8fl oz) almond milk or other milk

A few ice cubes

SERVES 1

233 calories per serving

Method

Place all of the ingredients into a blender and process until smooth.

Plum, Ginger & Beetroot Smoothie

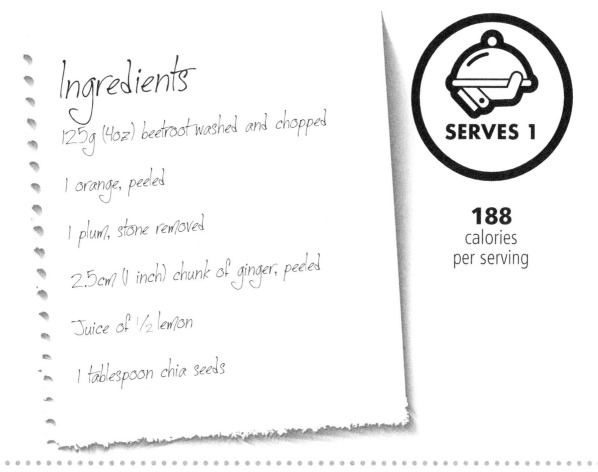

Ingredients

125g (4oz) beetroot washed and chopped

1 orange, peeled

1 plum, stone removed

2.5cm (1 inch) chunk of ginger, peeled

Juice of ½ lemon

1 tablespoon chia seeds

SERVES 1

188
calories
per serving

Method

Place the ingredients into a blender and add just enough water to cover them. Blitz until smooth. Drink straight away.

Pineapple & Lime Smoothie

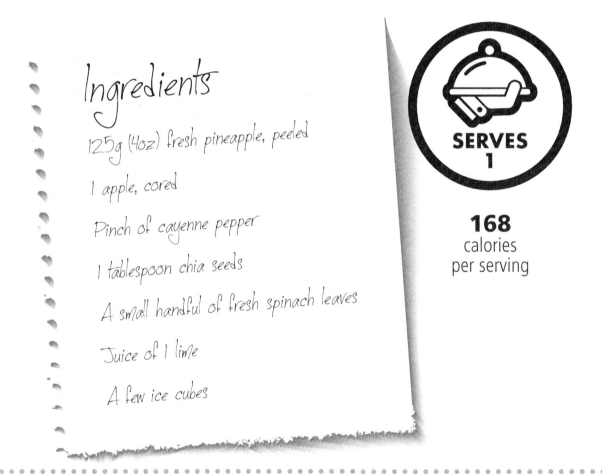

Ingredients

125g (4oz) fresh pineapple, peeled

1 apple, cored

Pinch of cayenne pepper

1 tablespoon chia seeds

A small handful of fresh spinach leaves

Juice of 1 lime

A few ice cubes

SERVES 1

168
calories
per serving

Method

Place all of the ingredients into the blender with enough cold water to cover them and blitz until smooth. Drink straight away.

Wheatgrass, Lemon & Ginger Smoothie

SERVES 1

64
calories
per serving

Ingredients

100g (3½ oz) honeydew melon flesh

1 teaspoon wheatgrass powder

Juice of ½ lemon

1cm (roughly ½ inch) chunk of ginger

1 teaspoon spirulina

A small handful of kale or spinach

Method

Place all of the ingredients into a blender and add enough water to cover them. Blitz until smooth. Drink straight away.

Hydrating Apple, Coriander & Chilli Smoothie

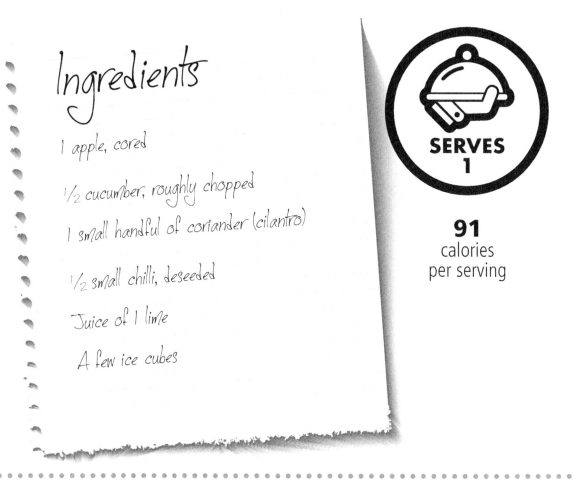

Ingredients

1 apple, cored

1/2 cucumber, roughly chopped

1 small handful of coriander (cilantro)

1/2 small chilli, deseeded

Juice of 1 lime

A few ice cubes

SERVES 1

91 calories per serving

Method

Place all of the ingredients into a blender with just enough water to cover them and blitz until smooth.

Detox Wheatgrass & Beetroot Smoothie

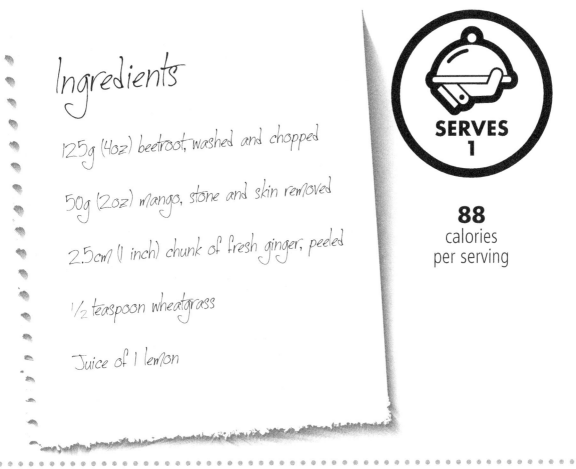

Ingredients

125g (4oz) beetroot, washed and chopped

50g (2oz) mango, stone and skin removed

2.5cm (1 inch) chunk of fresh ginger, peeled

½ teaspoon wheatgrass

Juice of 1 lemon

SERVES 1

88 calories per serving

Method

Place all of the ingredients into a blender and add enough water to cover them. Blitz until smooth. Drink straight away.

Pear, Grape & Lucuma Smoothie

Ingredients

125g (4oz) seedless grapes

1 tablespoons ground almonds

1 teaspoon lucuma powder

1/2 teaspoon cinnamon

1/2 teaspoon nutmeg

240mls (1/2 pint) almond milk (or other milk)

A small handful of spinach

A few ice cubes

SERVES 1

251 calories per serving

Method

Place all of the ingredients into a blitz until smooth and creamy. Garnish with a sprinkling of cinnamon and enjoy it straight away. This is a lovely smoothie with antioxidant and anti-inflammatory properties.

Lychee & Melon Smoothie

SERVES 1

147 calories per serving

Ingredients

125g (4oz) melon

125g (4oz) grapes

2 lychees, pitted and peeled

1cm (roughly ½ inch) fresh ginger root, peeled

1 teaspoon lucuma powder

A small handful of spinach

A few ice cubes

Method

Place all of the ingredients into a blender with enough water to cover them. Process until smooth and enjoy straight away.

Mango, Celery & Ginger Smoothie

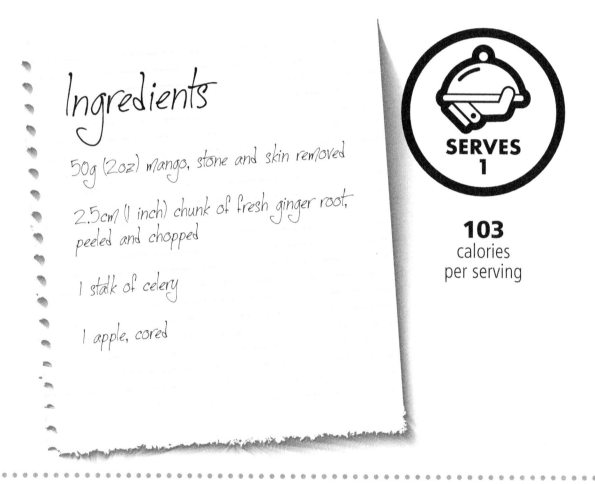

Ingredients

50g (2oz) mango, stone and skin removed

2.5cm (1 inch) chunk of fresh ginger root, peeled and chopped

1 stalk of celery

1 apple, cored

SERVES 1

103 calories per serving

Method

Put all the ingredients into a blender with some water and blitz until smooth. Add ice to make your smoothie really refreshing.

Orange, Carrot & Kale Smoothie

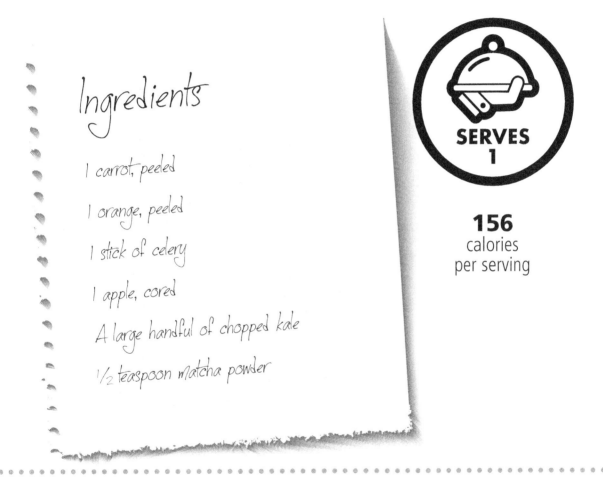

Ingredients

1 carrot, peeled

1 orange, peeled

1 stick of celery

1 apple, cored

A large handful of chopped kale

½ teaspoon matcha powder

SERVES 1

156 calories per serving

Method

Place all of the ingredients into a blender and add in enough water to cover them. Process until smooth, serve and enjoy.

Creamy Strawberry & Cherry Smoothie

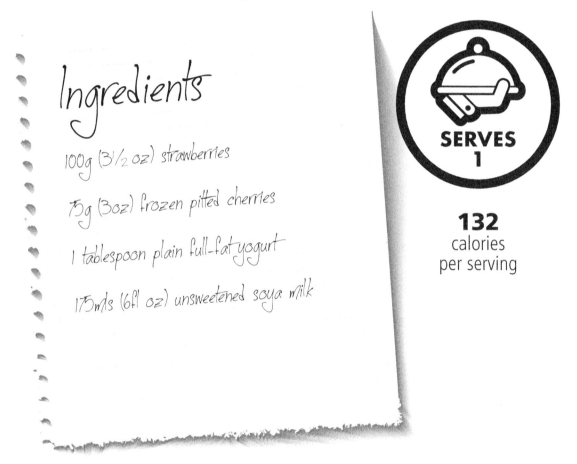

SERVES 1

132 calories per serving

Ingredients

100g (3½ oz) strawberries

75g (3oz) frozen pitted cherries

1 tablespoon plain full-fat yogurt

175mls (6fl oz) unsweetened soya milk

Method

Place all of the ingredients into a blender and process until smooth. Serve and enjoy.

Cranberry & Kale Crush

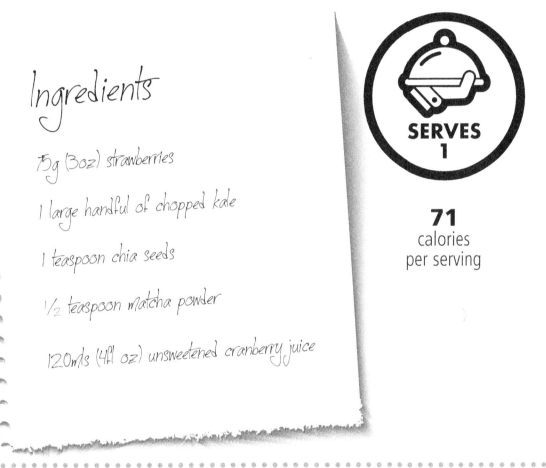

Ingredients

75g (3oz) strawberries

1 large handful of chopped kale

1 teaspoon chia seeds

1/2 teaspoon matcha powder

120mls (4fl oz) unsweetened cranberry juice

SERVES 1

71 calories per serving

Method

Place all of the ingredients into a blender and process until smooth. You can also add some crushed ice and a mint leaf or two for a really refreshing drink.

Mango & Rocket (Arugula) Smoothie

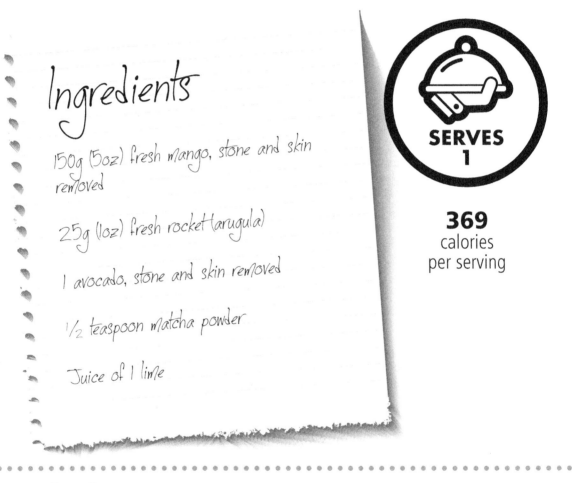

Ingredients

150g (5oz) fresh mango, stone and skin removed

25g (1oz) fresh rocket (arugula)

1 avocado, stone and skin removed

1/2 teaspoon matcha powder

Juice of 1 lime

SERVES 1

369 calories per serving

Method

Place all of the ingredients into a blender with enough water to cover them and process until smooth. Add a few ice cubes and enjoy.

Spiced Carrot Refresher

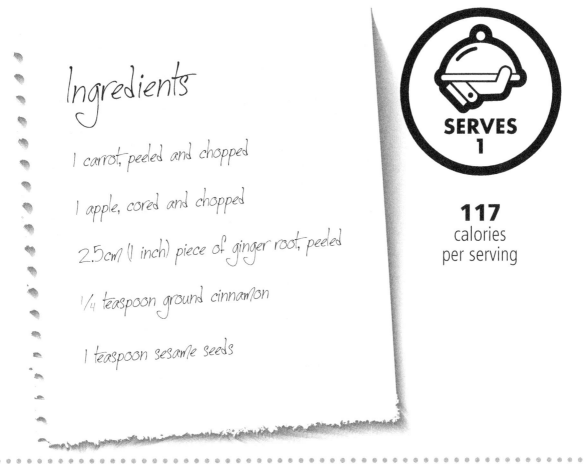

Ingredients

1 carrot, peeled and chopped

1 apple, cored and chopped

2.5cm (1 inch) piece of ginger root, peeled

1/4 teaspoon ground cinnamon

1 teaspoon sesame seeds

**SERVES
1**

117
calories
per serving

Method

Place all of the ingredients into a blender with enough water to cover them. Blitz until smooth. Serve and drink straight away.

Berry & Carrot Smoothie

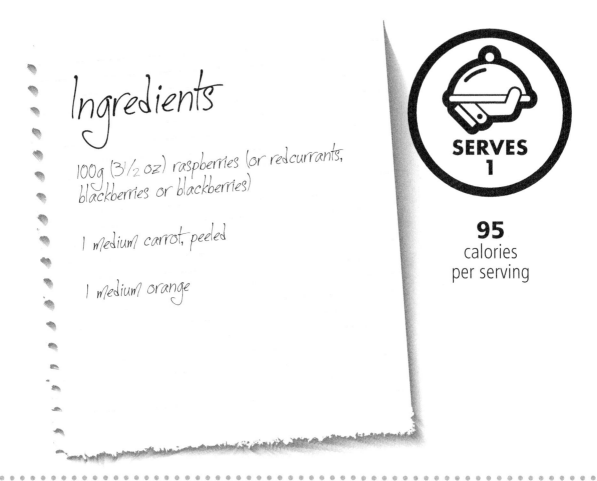

SERVES 1

95 calories per serving

Ingredients

100g (3½ oz) raspberries (or redcurrants, blackberries or blackberries)

1 medium carrot, peeled

1 medium orange

Method

Place all the ingredients into a blender with enough water to cover them and process until smooth. Serve and enjoy.

Coconut, Spinach & Lime Smoothie

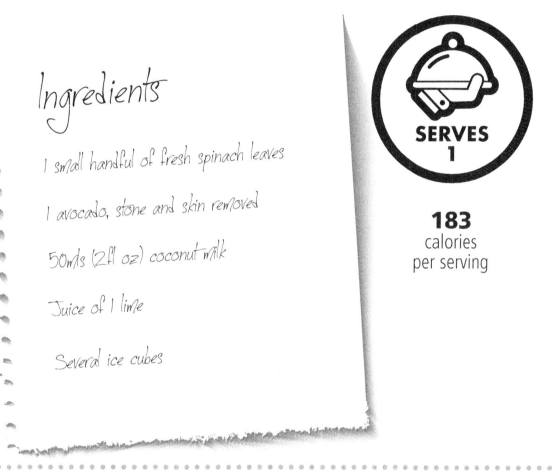

Ingredients

1 small handful of fresh spinach leaves

1 avocado, stone and skin removed

50mls (2fl oz) coconut milk

Juice of 1 lime

Several ice cubes

SERVES 1

183 calories per serving

Method

Place all of the ingredients into a food processor and add just enough water to cover them. Blitz until smooth and creamy. Serve and drink straight away.

Cleansing Cucumber Smoothie

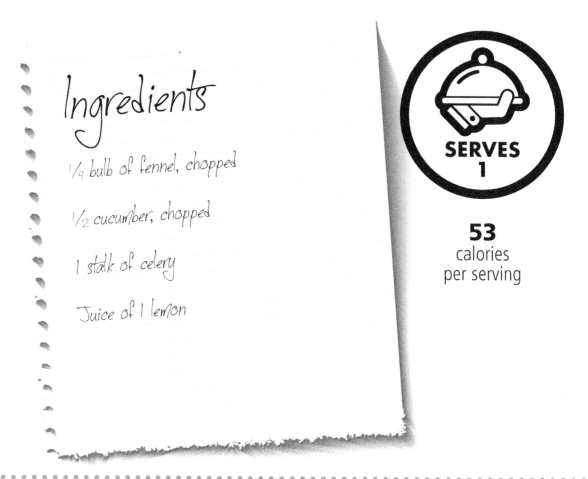

Ingredients

1/4 bulb of fennel, chopped

1/2 cucumber, chopped

1 stalk of celery

Juice of 1 lemon

SERVES 1

53 calories per serving

Method

Place the fennel, cucumber and celery into a food processor or smoothie maker and add the lemon juice together with enough water to cover the ingredients. Process until smooth.

Minty Lime Shots

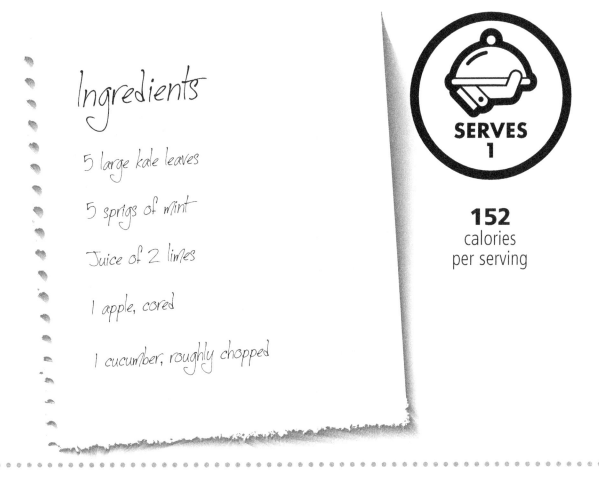

Ingredients

5 large kale leaves

5 sprigs of mint

Juice of 2 limes

1 apple, cored

1 cucumber, roughly chopped

SERVES 1

152 calories per serving

Method

Place the ingredients into a blender and add sufficient water to cover the ingredients. Store in a bottle in the fridge and take healthy shots throughout the day or you can just drink it all straight away.

Chocolate Protein Shake

Ingredients

2 teaspoons vanilla whey protein powder (sugar-free)

1 teaspoon 100% cocoa powder

1 teaspoon peanut butter

1/4 teaspoon stevia sweetener (optional)

200mls (7fl oz) unsweetened almond milk

Several ice cubes

SERVES 1

115 calories per serving

Method

Place all of the ingredients into blender or food processor and blitz until smooth. Serve into a glass and enjoy!

Kiwi & Lettuce Shots

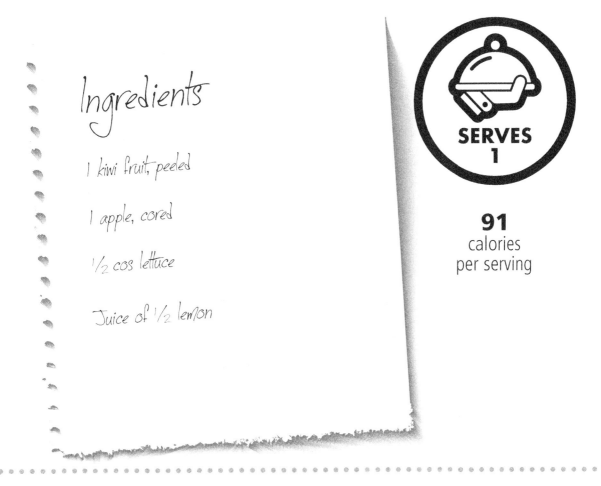

Ingredients

1 kiwi fruit, peeled

1 apple, cored

½ cos lettuce

Juice of ½ lemon

SERVES 1

91 calories per serving

Method

Place all of the ingredients into a food processor with just enough water to cover them. Blitz until smooth. Pour the liquid into a glass bottle and keep it in the fridge, ready for you to have fresh shots throughout the day. Alternatively you can just drink it all straight away.

Pear Salad Smoothie

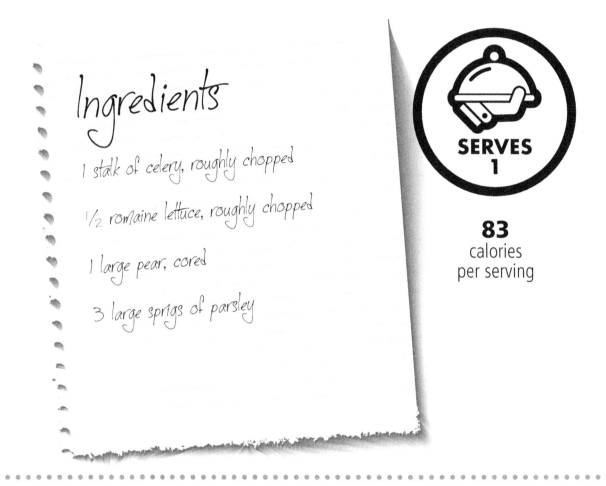

Ingredients

1 stalk of celery, roughly chopped

½ romaine lettuce, roughly chopped

1 large pear, cored

3 large sprigs of parsley

SERVES
1

83
calories
per serving

Method

Place all of the ingredients into a blender with sufficient water to cover them and blitz until smooth.

Avocado & Banana Smoothie

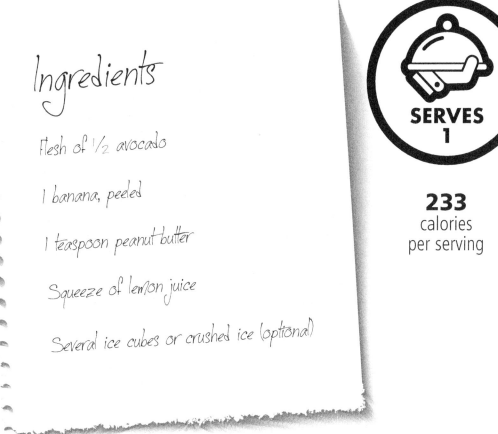

SERVES 1

233 calories per serving

Ingredients

Flesh of 1/2 avocado

1 banana, peeled

1 teaspoon peanut butter

Squeeze of lemon juice

Several ice cubes or crushed ice (optional)

Method

Place all of the ingredients into a blender and blitz until smooth. If your blender doesn't tolerate ice you can just add a few cubes for serving.

Pear & Cucumber Smoothie

SERVES 1

212 calories per serving

Ingredients

3 sprigs of parsley

1 pear, cored

1 tablespoon ground almonds (almond meal/ almond flour)

½ cucumber

A large handful of fresh spinach leaves

Method

Place all of the ingredients into a blender and process until smooth. Drink straight away.

Cucumber, Lemon & Coconut Refresher

SERVES 1

124 calories per serving

Ingredients

A large handful of lettuce leaves

1 apple, cored

1/4 cucumber

Juice of 1/2 lemon

250mls (8fl oz) coconut water

Method

Place all of the ingredients into a blender and blitz until smooth. Serve straight away.

Pink Grapefruit & Turmeric Smoothie

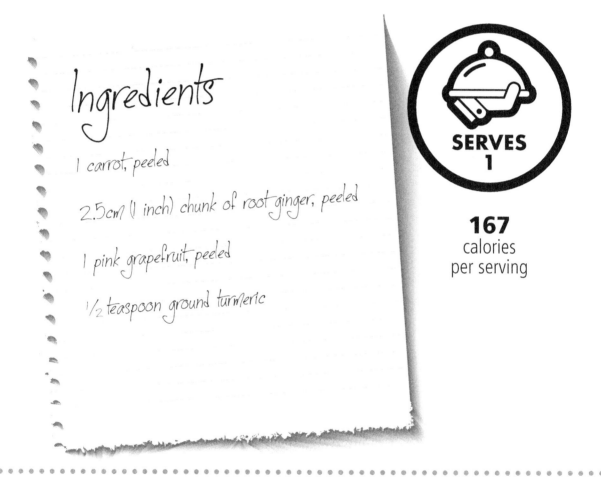

SERVES 1

167 calories per serving

Ingredients

1 carrot, peeled

2.5cm (1 inch) chunk of root ginger, peeled

1 pink grapefruit, peeled

1/2 teaspoon ground turmeric

Method

Place all of the ingredients into a blender with sufficient water to just cover the ingredients. Blitz until smooth. Serve with a few ice cubes and enjoy.

Peanut Butter & Banana Smoothie

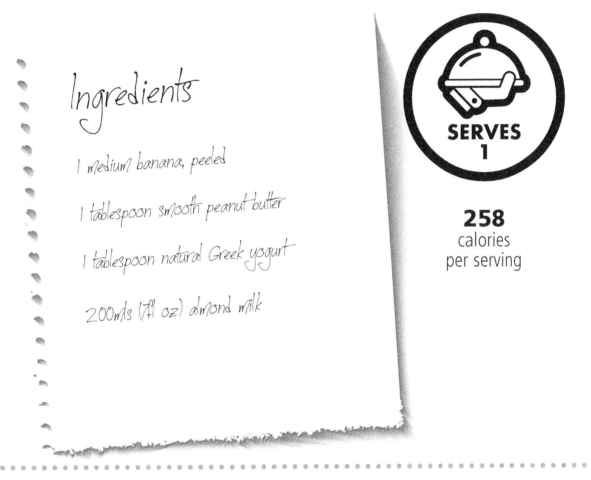

Ingredients

1 medium banana, peeled

1 tablespoon smooth peanut butter

1 tablespoon natural Greek yogurt

200mls (7fl oz) almond milk

**SERVES
1**

258
calories
per serving

Method

Place all the ingredients into a blender and process until smooth and creamy. Serve with a few ice cubes and drink straight away.

Carrot & Celery Cleanser

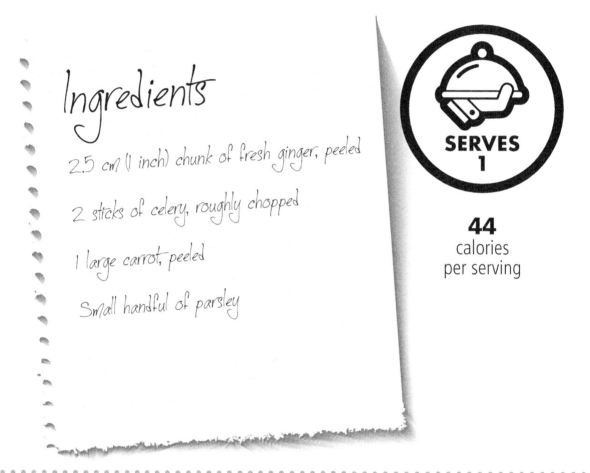

Ingredients

2.5 cm (1 inch) chunk of fresh ginger, peeled

2 sticks of celery, roughly chopped

1 large carrot, peeled

Small handful of parsley

SERVES 1

44 calories per serving

Method

Place all of the ingredients into a blender and blitz until smooth.

Nutty Kale Smoothie

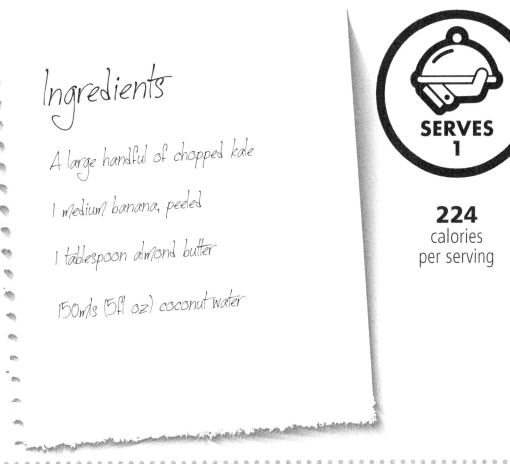

SERVES 1

224 calories per serving

Ingredients

A large handful of chopped kale

1 medium banana, peeled

1 tablespoon almond butter

150mls (5fl oz) coconut water

Method

Place all of the ingredients in a blender and process until smooth.

Tomato & Ginger Smoothie

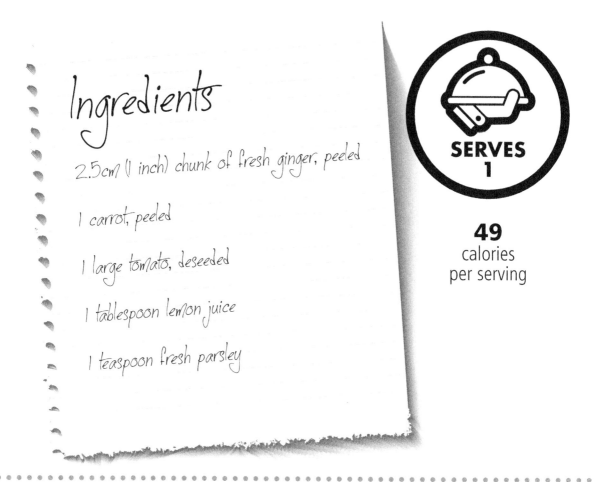

Ingredients

2.5cm (1 inch) chunk of fresh ginger, peeled

1 carrot, peeled

1 large tomato, deseeded

1 tablespoon lemon juice

1 teaspoon fresh parsley

SERVES 1

49 calories per serving

Method

Place all of the ingredients into a blender with just enough water to cover them. Blitz until smooth. Serve with ice cubes.

Grapefruit & Carrot Smoothie

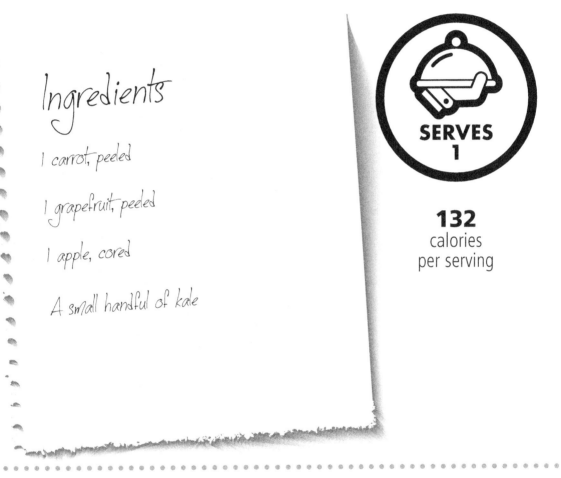

Ingredients

1 carrot, peeled

1 grapefruit, peeled

1 apple, cored

A small handful of kale

SERVES 1

132 calories per serving

Method

Place all of the ingredients into a blender and process until smooth.

Coffee & Almond Smoothie

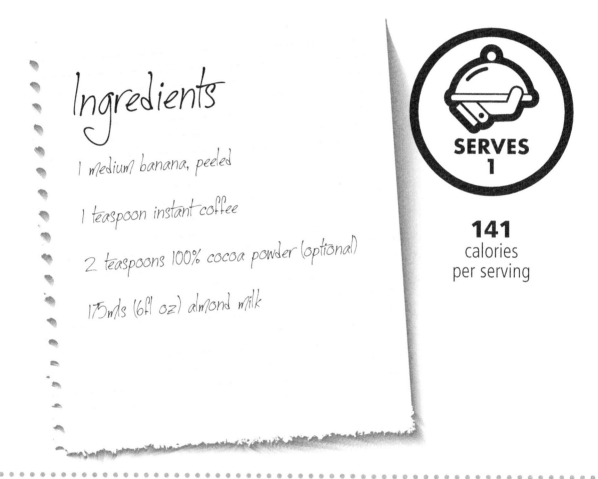

Ingredients

1 medium banana, peeled

1 teaspoon instant coffee

2 teaspoons 100% cocoa powder (optional)

175mls (6fl oz) almond milk

SERVES 1

141 calories per serving

Method

Place all of the ingredients into a blender and process until smooth. Serve with a few ice cubes.

Banana & Coconut Smoothie

Ingredients

1 medium banana, peeled

2 tablespoons plain (unflavoured) Greek yogurt

75mls (3fl oz) coconut milk

75mls (3fl oz) water

**SERVES
1**

317
calories
per serving

Method

Toss all the ingredients into a blender and blitz. Pour and enjoy!

Basil Blackcurrant Refresher

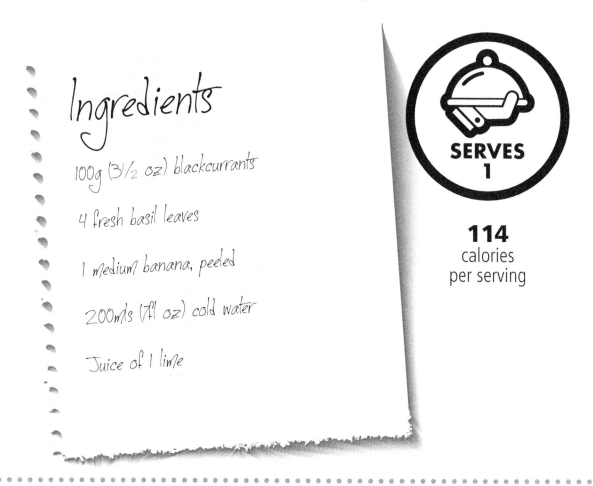

Ingredients

100g (3½ oz) blackcurrants

4 fresh basil leaves

1 medium banana, peeled

200mls (7fl oz) cold water

Juice of 1 lime

**SERVES
1**

114
calories
per serving

Method

Place all of the ingredients into a blender and process until smooth. Drink straight away or keep it in the fridge and take little 'shots' throughout the day.

Kiwi & Coconut Smoothie

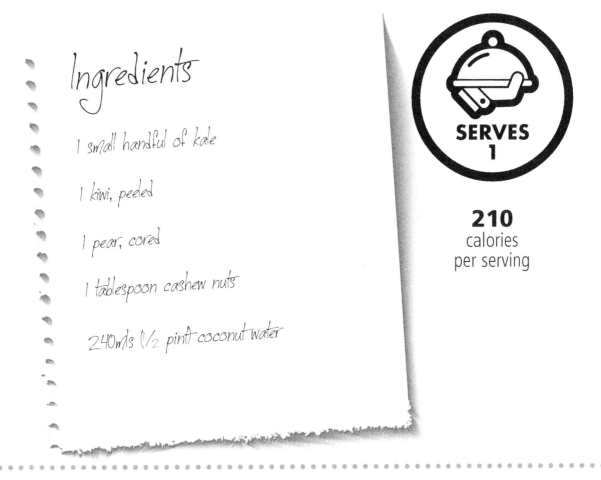

Ingredients

1 small handful of kale

1 kiwi, peeled

1 pear, cored

1 tablespoon cashew nuts

240mls (½ pint) coconut water

SERVES 1

210 calories per serving

Method

Place all of the ingredients into a blender and process until smooth. Serve and drink straight away.

Lush Green Smoothie

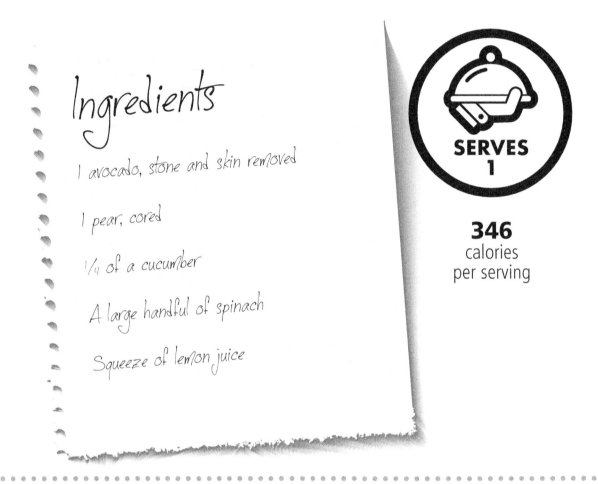

Ingredients

1 avocado, stone and skin removed

1 pear, cored

1/4 of a cucumber

A large handful of spinach

Squeeze of lemon juice

SERVES 1

346 calories per serving

Method

Place all of the ingredients into a blender and add just enough water to cover them. Blitz until smooth and creamy. Serve and drink immediately

Apple, Spinach & Seed Smoothie

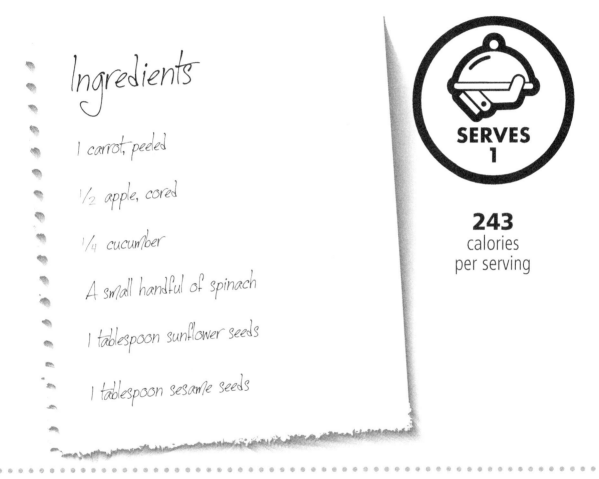

Ingredients

1 carrot, peeled

1/2 apple, cored

1/4 cucumber

A small handful of spinach

1 tablespoon sunflower seeds

1 tablespoon sesame seeds

SERVES 1

243 calories per serving

Method

Place all the ingredients into a blender and add around a cup of water. Blitz until smooth. You can add a little extra water if it's too thick.

Coconut & Cucumber Smoothie

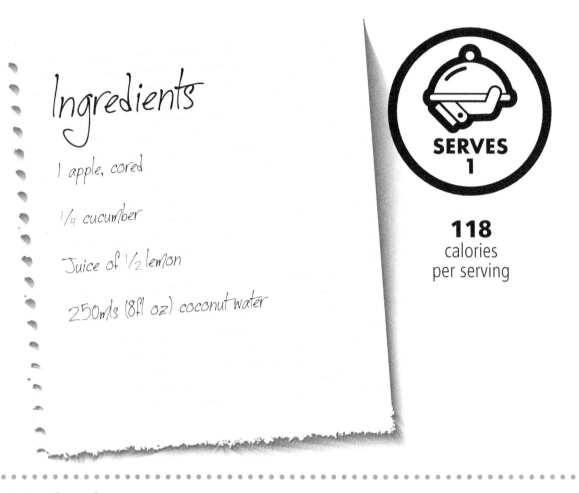

Ingredients

1 apple, cored

¼ cucumber

Juice of ½ lemon

250mls (8fl oz) coconut water

SERVES 1

118 calories per serving

Method

Place all of the ingredients into a blender and blitz until smooth. Serve straight away.

Green Detox Smoothie

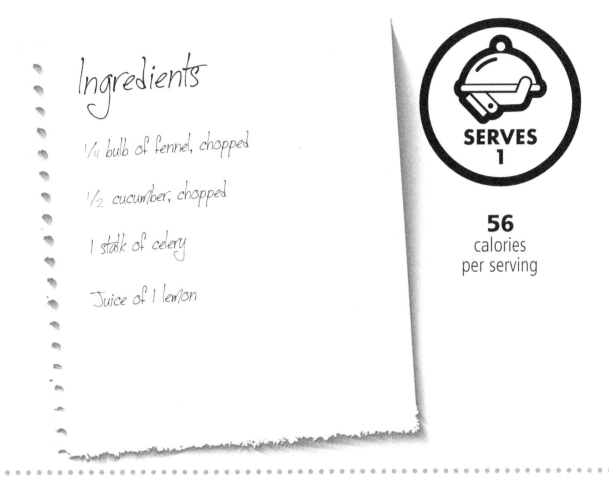

Ingredients

1/4 bulb of fennel, chopped

1/2 cucumber, chopped

1 stalk of celery

Juice of 1 lemon

SERVES 1

56 calories per serving

Method

Place the all of the ingredients into a food processor or smoothie maker and pour in enough water to cover the ingredients. Process until smooth.

Raspberry & Carrot Smoothie

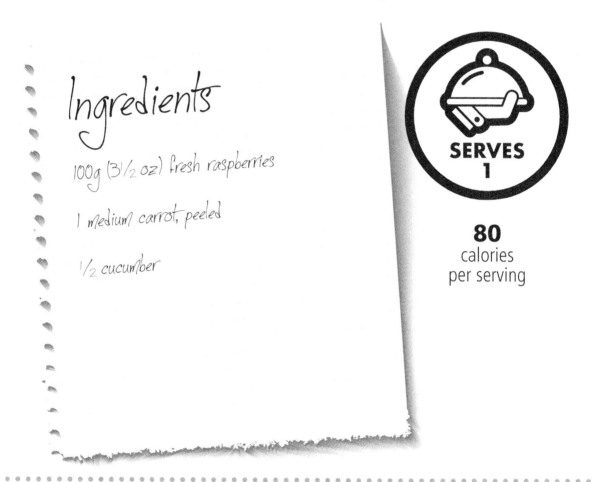

Ingredients

100g (3½ oz) fresh raspberries

1 medium carrot, peeled

½ cucumber

**SERVES
1**

80
calories
per serving

Method

Place the ingredients into a blender with enough water to cover it and process until smooth.

Tomato & Carrot Smoothie

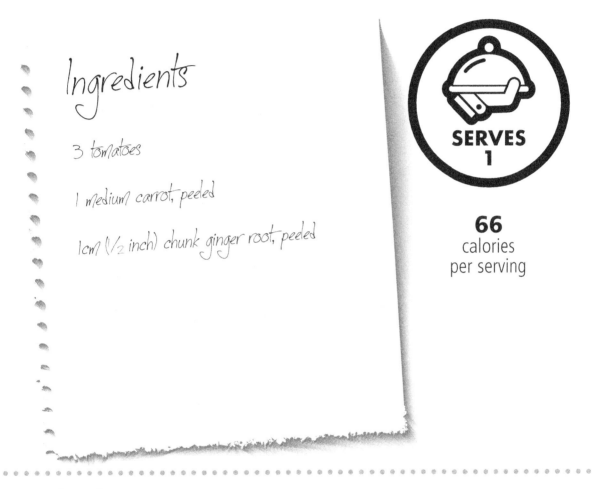

Ingredients

3 tomatoes

1 medium carrot, peeled

1cm (½ inch) chunk ginger root, peeled

SERVES 1

66 calories per serving

Method

Place the ingredients into a blender with sufficient water to cover them. Blitz until smooth.

Apple & Grapefruit Smoothie

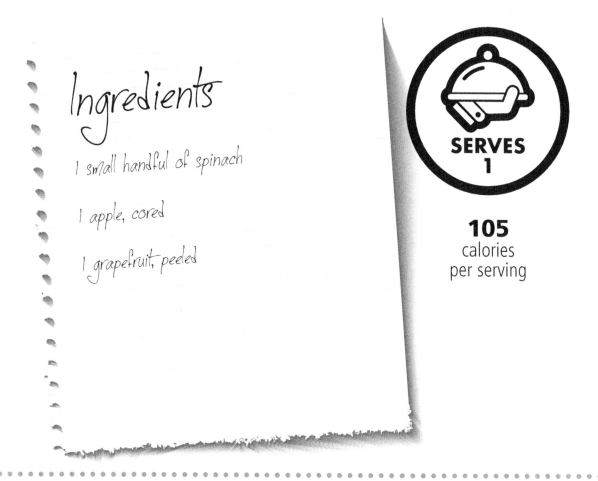

Ingredients

1 small handful of spinach

1 apple, cored

1 grapefruit, peeled

SERVES 1

105 calories per serving

Method

Place all the ingredients into a blender with enough water to cover them and blitz until smooth.

Cashew & Apricot Smoothie

Ingredients

SERVES 1

249 calories per serving

25g (1oz) unsalted cashew nuts

1 medium banana, peeled

1 apricot, stone removed

225mls (8fl oz) unsweetened almond milk

Method

Place all of the ingredients into a blender and process until smooth. Serve and drink straight away.

Carrot & Apple Smoothie

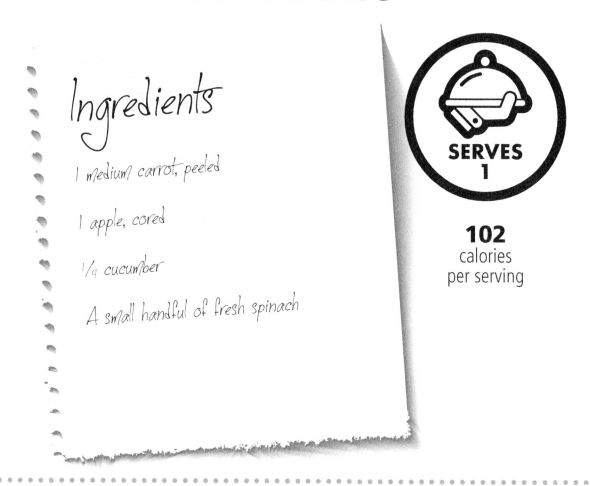

Ingredients

1 medium carrot, peeled

1 apple, cored

1/4 cucumber

A small handful of fresh spinach

SERVES 1

102 calories per serving

Method

Place all the ingredients into a blender with just enough water to cover them. Blitz until smooth. Enjoy.

Apple & Ginger Smoothie

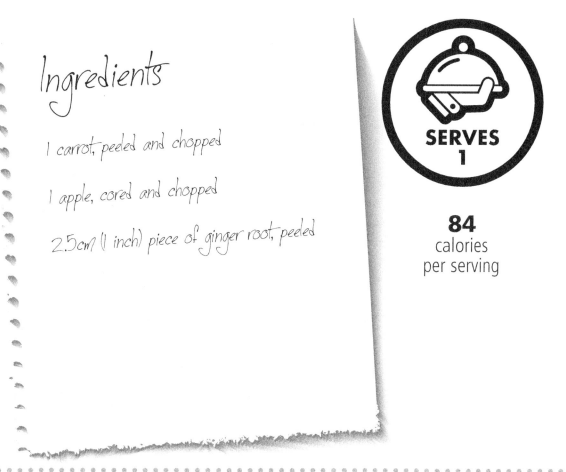

Ingredients

1 carrot, peeled and chopped

1 apple, cored and chopped

2.5cm (1 inch) piece of ginger root, peeled

SERVES 1

84 calories per serving

Method

Place all of the ingredients into a blender with enough water to cover them. Blitz until smooth. Serve and drink straight away.

Detox Smoothie

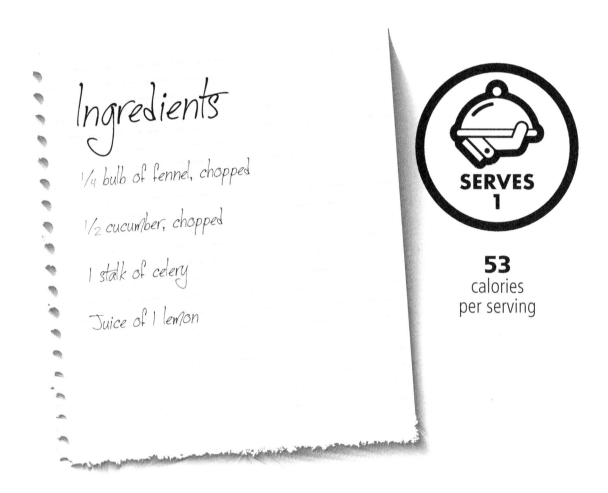

Ingredients

¼ bulb of fennel, chopped

½ cucumber, chopped

1 stalk of celery

Juice of 1 lemon

**SERVES
1**

53
calories
per serving

Method

Place the fennel, cucumber and celery into a food processor or smoothie maker and add the lemon juice together with enough water to cover the ingredients. Process until smooth. Drink straight away.

Carrot & Blackberry Smoothie

Ingredients

100g (3½ oz) blackberries

1 medium carrot, peeled

1 medium orange, peeled

Pinch of cinnamon

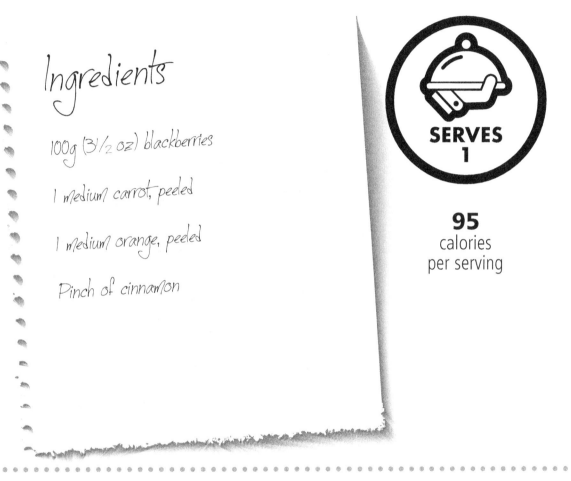

SERVES 1

95 calories per serving

Method

Place all the ingredients into a blender with enough water to cover them and process until smooth.

Kiwi Salad Smoothie

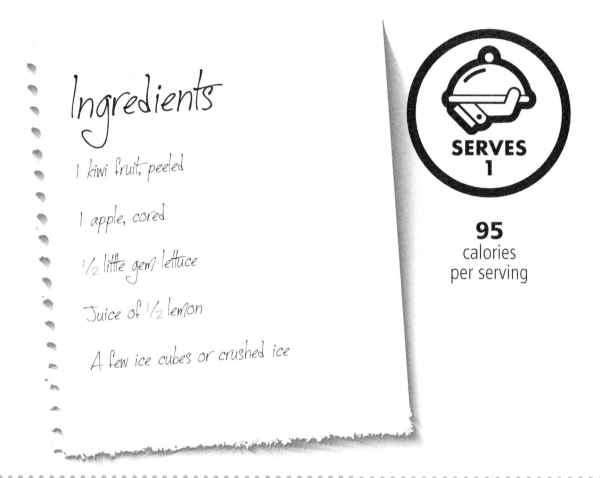

Ingredients

1 kiwi fruit, peeled

1 apple, cored

1/2 little gem lettuce

Juice of 1/2 lemon

A few ice cubes or crushed ice

SERVES 1

95 calories per serving

Method

Place all of the ingredients into a food processor with just enough water to cover them. Blitz until smooth. If your blender can't process ice cubes just add them to the glass. Drink straight away.

Blackberry & Carrot Smoothie

Ingredients

100g (3½ oz) blackberries

1 medium carrot, peeled

1 medium orange, peeled

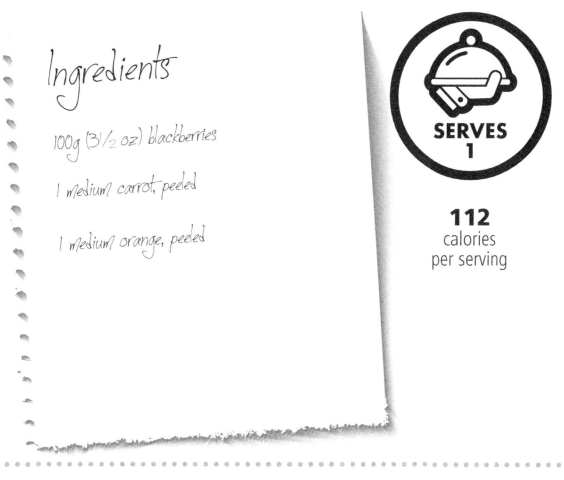

SERVES 1

112 calories per serving

Method

Place all the ingredients into a blender with enough water to cover them and process until smooth. Serve and drink straight away.

Coconut & Lemon Zinger

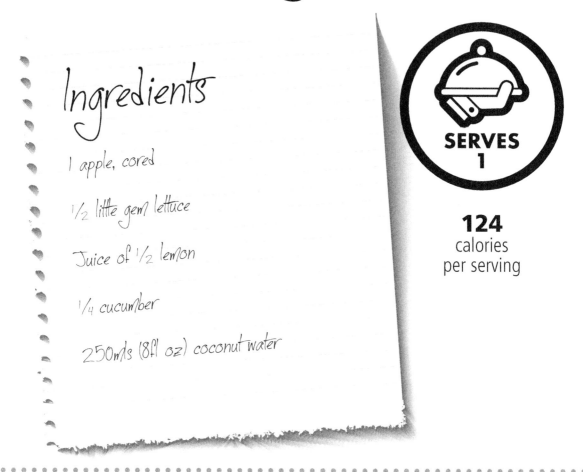

SERVES 1

124 calories per serving

Ingredients

1 apple, cored

½ little gem lettuce

Juice of ½ lemon

¼ cucumber

250mls (8fl oz) coconut water

Method

Place all of the ingredients into a blender and blitz until smooth. Serve straight away.

Creamy Raspberry Smoothie

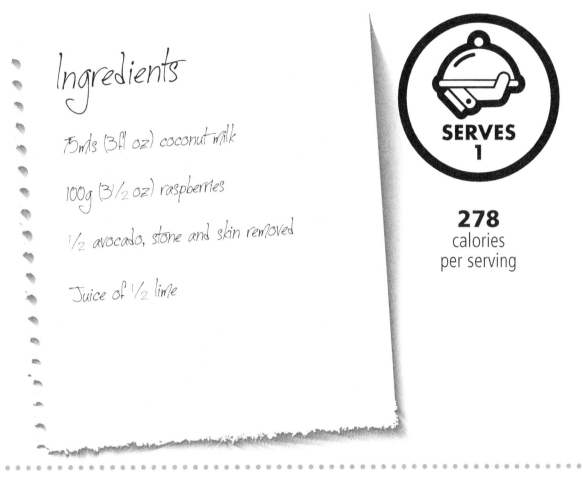

Ingredients

75mls (3fl oz) coconut milk

100g (3½ oz) raspberries

½ avocado, stone and skin removed

Juice of ½ lime

**SERVES
1**

278
calories
per serving

Method

Toss all of the ingredients into a blender. Blitz until smooth and creamy. If it seems too thick you can add some water. Pour and enjoy!

You may also be interested in other titles by
Erin Rose Publishing
which are available in both paperback and ebook.

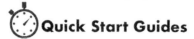 Quick Start Guides

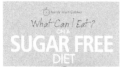
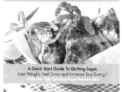
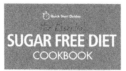
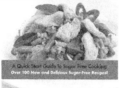
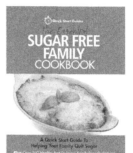
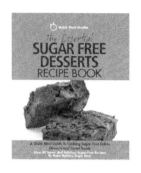

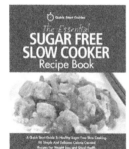
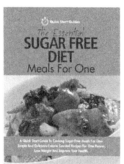
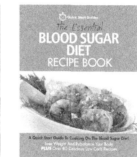
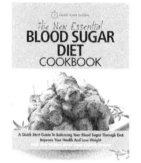

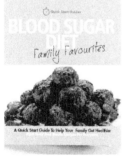
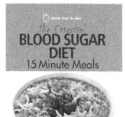
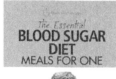
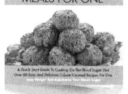
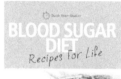
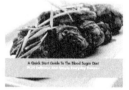

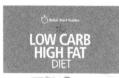
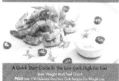
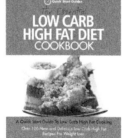
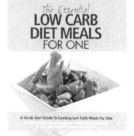
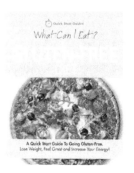